The Herpes Solution

How To Free Yourself from Genital Herpes… for Good!

Angie S

Limits of Liability, Disclaimer of Warranties & Terms of Use
This book is a general educational health-related information product. As an express condition to reading this book, you understand and agree to following terms. The information and advice contained in this book are not intended as a substitute for consulting with a healthcare professional.

The publisher and authors are not responsible for any adverse effects or consequences resulting from the use of any of the suggestions, or procedures discussed in this book. While all attempts have been made to verify information provided in this book, the author and publisher assume no responsibility for errors, omissions, or contrary interpretation of the subject matter herein. All matters pertaining to your physical health should be supervised by a health care professional

ISBN: 1499539592
ISBN-13: 978-1499539592

DEDICATION

For those in search of a reliable and effective genital herpes solution.

CONTENTS

INTRODUCTION

I want to thank you for purchasing this book, "The Genital Herpes Solution".

This book contains vital information about genital herpes and the proper procedures needed to get rid of it. If you are one of the many people that suffer from genital herpes, you may be wondering exactly what it will take to get rid of the embarrassing virus

Although I know that this is not, in any shape or form, a popular subject to talk about. I realized that there are plenty of people going through the same situation, so my goal is to lead you in the right direction towards finding that solution.

CHAPTER 1 - THE BASICS ABOUT GENITAL HERPES

Genital herpes is one of the most common sexually transmitted diseases (STD). It is viral in nature and is caused by a virus called herpes simplex virus or HSV. As of 2013, genital herpes is the most common STD if we are to consider the number of the reported cases.

The Herpes Simplex Virus

Herpes simplex virus or HSV is a virus from the Herpesviradae family which basically infects humans. The HSV is also known as human herpesvirus 1 and 2 (HHV 1 and HHV2).

HHV1 and HHV2 are the two types of herpes simplex virus. Both viruses are widespread viruses and can infect others upon contact. The difference between 1 and 2 are the common sites of their infections. HHV1 is commonly seen around the mouth as cold sores; while HHV2 is the herpes virus that causes most of the genital herpes.

The most common symptom of both viruses is the formation of watery blisters around the mouth, lips or genitalia. When healed, these blisters will become scabbed lesions.

Often, herpes are mild and atypical. However, the virus never leave the nerves of the body, staying there until they will be triggered again for the next outbreak which causes new sores to appear.

Herpes Genitalis

Herpes genitalis or most commonly known as genital herpes is an infection that affects the genital area of both male and female patients. It is a sexually transmitted disease and it passes on to other by skin contact or body fluid transfers.

Herpes genitalis was once caused by HSV 2 only, however, recently, due to the rising incidence of younger people engaged in sexual activities, genital herpes that is caused by HSV1 has become surprisingly common. As a matter of fact, almost 80% of genital herpes incidences are caused by HSV1.

As with any infection caused by herpes, the symptom of genital herpes is the formation of blisters around the genital area of the infected person. In males, the glans penis and anus are infected while affected females have blisters around their vaginal area near the pubis, clitoris, vulva and anus.

There is really no cure for genital herpes; although the virus will become dormant overtime, it will still stay in the patient's system and "live" in their nerves. When activated, the virus will travel from the nerves to the site of the infected area. This is where the virus will replicate itself.

The process of replication or copying oneself is typically called shedding. It is so called as such because the replicated viruses now have the ability to infect other people simply by rubbing the infected area to the skin.

After the outbreak, the virus will then travel from the site of infection back to the patient's nerves. It will find a ganglion (a mass of nerve tissue usually found at the base of the spine) and becomes dormant again until the next activation.

The Spread of Genital Herpes

As stated, genital herpes is transmitted from one person to another via direct contact. This contact can be kissing; oral, vaginal or anal sex; or skin to skin contact.

Although commonly identified from the presence of blistery sores, it can still be transmitted with or without these indications. In fact, genital herpes is often transferred by people with asymptomatic herpes not knowing that they are already infected.

Genital Herpes Statistics

Genital herpes is considered to be the most common sexually transmitted disease according to the currently reported cases. In the United States alone, almost 45 million people are infected with HSV-2. Their ages range from 12 onwards with a ratio of one out of five from the total population of adolescents and adults.

The infection is more commonly recorded in women than with males. They are attributing this to the more efficient transmission of the disease from male to female than the other way around.

Among the races, herpes genitalis is also more prevalent in African Americans than with Caucasians; however, it may not be racial alone. It could also be attributed to other health determinants like poverty, access to health care and medicines, drug-use and contaminated living quarters.

The disease is also seen to be increasing. A 30% increase has been recorded from 1978-79. The increased rate was said to be caused by the disease's prevalence in young white teens.

The Seriousness of Herpes Genitalis

Normally, genital herpes is a disease with very mild symptoms. There are even some instances when the infection has no symptoms at all. However, in some cases, the herpes simplex virus 2 or HSV2 can cause painful ulcers that recur over and over again. More severe symptoms can even be expected from people who have compromised immune systems.

However, STD such as herpes genitalia inflicts more than physical symptoms. It is important to note that patients who have been diagnosed with genital herpes, no matter how mild or how severe their symptoms are, will be distressed psychologically.

Sadly, there are also some instances that the HSV2 can be fatal. Infants who are born with mothers who are shedding on their birth date have a big chance of fatally contracting the disease. Because of this, it is very important for women to avoid getting the infection at any cost.

In addition to such serious complications, it has also been reported in the United States that HSV2 makes the infected patient more susceptible to the AIDS' virus – HIV.

CHAPTER 2 - THE DIFFERENT SYMPTOMS OF GENITAL HERPES

Genital herpes is caused by the herpes simplex virus 1 and 2. It is passed on from one person to another through direct contact. Kissing and sexual intercourse are two of the most common contacts that bring the infection. Among the two herpes simplex viruses, the HSV2 is the one that usually causes genital herpes, however, HSV1 has been lately causing more than cold sores, as well.

The virus will enter the system through the skin, then it will roam along inside the body through the paths provided by the nerves. It will then attach itself in a nerve ganglion or a mass of nerve tissue where it will remain dormant or inactive unless it will be activated.

During activation, the herpes virus will travel back again from the ganglion to the surface of the skin where it will replicate itself in a process called shedding. This replication may cause an outbreak of symptoms to appear or it may simply remain asymptomatic, although still very contagious. It is interesting to note that a condom cannot really save one partner from the other because the herpes virus can very well infect with the exposed portion of the skin.

Transmission in Women and Men

Women are 4 times more likely to get the herpes type 2 virus than men. Women that are vulnerable are more likely to contract genital herpes from an infected man than if it were the other way around. Meaning, if a non-infected man and woman were to have intercourse with someone who is infected, the likelihood of the woman contracting the herpes virus is greater than the man.

The reasons for which women are more vulnerable to genital herpes infection are:

- The genital area has a greater surface area of cells moist with body fluids (mucosal cells) than men.
- Hormone changes during a woman's menstrual cycle may affect the immune system, making it easier for the herpes simplex virus to cause an infection.

The Symptoms of Genital Herpes

Symptoms may or may not appear upon the onset of infection. If it will, then it will be characterized by the following symptoms:

1. Reddish skin that is cracked or raw along the genital area. This will not cause any pain or itching or tingling sensation
2. Itching or tingling sensation around the genitalia or anal region.
3. Sores brought by painful blisters breaking open. These sores can be seen around the vagina, penis,

anus or thighs. There are also some reported cases of blisters occurring at the urethra which will cause severe pain when urine is being transported through here.

4. Headaches and chilling as a reaction to the infection
5. Backaches
6. Fever
7. Swollen lymph nodes
8.

Even with all of these symptoms present, one cannot still be sure if he contracted genital herpes. These signs can also be the characteristics of other sexually transmitted diseases like vaginal yeast infection or bladder infections.

In order to accurately identify which one had infected the person, it is best to undergo some tests under the facilitation and management of a physician or specialist.

Herpes Outbreaks

The first episode of herpes genitalis is often the most severe. It can last for weeks then it will retreat to the nerves to "live" there. It will be dormant unless triggered to be activated again.

It is normal that an outbreak will again recur weeks or months after the first episode. It is most probable that the recurrence will now be less severe than the first and it will probably last shorter than the first one ever did. After this, it will again retreat back to the nerves.

Please remember that the herpes virus stays in the human system forever. Fortunately, it has been observed that along the years, the outbreaks tend to be shorter, becoming less severe and less frequent as compared from the previous episodes.

The outbreak of the virus is naturally dependent on the infected person. It can be considered normal if a person will experience around 4 outbreaks in a year, with a gradual reduction in pain and severity after each outbreak incidence.

The triggers of the outbreaks are also dependent on the infected person's cases. The most common triggers are observed to be the following:

- Stress
- Compromised immune system
- Surgery
- Vigorous sexual activity
- Diet
- Menstrual period

The Herpes Virus and the Eyes

As it had been discussed, genital herpes nowadays can also be acquired from HSV1 and not by HSV2 alone.

It may be surprising to most people that HSV1, and the herpes virus responsible for chicken pox, can both cause herpetic eye disease. The eye infection is called herpes zoster opthalmicus. This eye condition cannot be transmitted through sexual intercourse. On the other hand, if the infection affects the cornea, the condition is now called as herpes simplex keratitis.

Both diseases have different symptoms, although both can be very careful. Two of the symptoms they share are the redness of the eye and the pain around one eye only. However, with herpes simplex keratitis, there is the presence of dirt and grit in the eye, overflowing tears, bright light avoidance because of pain and optic swelling.
As per treating herpetic eyes, it will be a waste to add any

antibiotics. It is not a bacterial infection but instead it is viral. Thus, the only thing that will help is an anti-viral medication.

CHAPTER 3 - DIAGNOSIS AND TESTS FOR GENITAL HERPES

No matter how common genital herpes is, the number of cases reported is still thought to be inaccurate. It is thought that more people are expected to be infected yet not all of these cases will be consulted and treated. Why? It is because genital herpes is oftentimes asymptomatic.

Many people who are carriers are not aware that they are infected because no symptom was ever felt or experienced. On the other hand, if the symptoms did occur, it can be easily mistaken for other diseases.

In order to be sure if you are carrying the virus or not, it is best to have yourself tested for HSV1 or 2. The genital herpes tests are the following:

1. PCR Blood Test

PCR blood test is a very accurate blood test which determines the nature of the virus by simply identifying it through the virus' DNA pieces. This test is also effective even if the patient is not exhibiting any symptoms from the infection.

2. Cell Culture

Cell culture is a process in which the physician will get a cell or tissue sample from the patient's sores and look up for the presence of HSV2 virus under the microscope.

Either of these tests can yield a negative result if the sores are already scabbed or if you are only carrying the infection very recently. The virus' antibodies will be able to register in the blood for several weeks after the contamination.

The results of these diagnostic tests can be:

a. False-negative: of the tests resulted to a negative condition when in fact you are truly infected
b. False-positive: your test results showed positive even if you don't have any of the virus' presence. If there is a little chance that you will get infected, get yourself retested in order to accurately identify your status.
c. Negative
d. Positive

Both tests are designed to tell you that you have been exposed to the virus on some point; neither can actually tell the exact time of contamination or onset of infection.

Other Tests

There are still some available diagnostic tests that one can use aside from the PCR blood tests and cellular tests, the two most common diagnostic tools for HSV.

An antibody test is one option.

As you know, antibodies are proteins that are being produced by our immune system whenever there is a presence of infection. The production is done to enable our body to fight the infection.

The antibody test designed for the identification of HSV is called Direct Fluorescent Antibody Test. Here, a solution mixed with HSV antibody and a fluorescent dye is dropped in cell sample. If the presence of HSV has been detected in the cell sample, the antibody will stick to the virus and glow. The glow of the dye will be visible if it will be placed and checked under a specialized microscope.

The good thing about the antibody test is its ability to differentiate HSV1 from HSV2. Knowing what herpes virus you have is important in gauging the frequency of your symptom outbreaks. HSV2 has been observed to be more frequent while HSV1 has lower incidences of outbreaks.

However, the test would not be able to tell you the specific onset of the outbreak. It is very limited to provide the information of the virus type and not the outbreak schedule.

There are other tests that are currently in the research pipeline. These tests are designed to identify the virus infection by inspecting the urine and saliva samples of the patient.

CHAPTER 4 - TREATMENT AND CARE FOR GENITAL HERPES PATIENTS

The first thing that you need to know is that there is no cure for herpes. Once infected, the virus lives in your nerves where it will remain dormant until the next virus activation. Fortunately, the severity of the symptom outbreaks seems to decrease as the years pass.

If you have been diagnosed with the infection and you are currently experiencing the worst of symptoms, there are treatments available in order to control them or shorten its duration. It may not be a cure but it will surely make your life a lot easier.

Currently, there are three drugs that are most prescribed by specialists. These are:

1. Acyclovir (Zovirax)

Acyclovir is an ethical drug used to treat the infections caused by certain herpes virus such as cold sores, chickenpox or shingles. This drug is also indicated to treat the symptoms of genital herpes' outbreak.

It decreases the severity of the outbreaks and shortens the duration of each one. Aside from these, acyclovir has been observed to aid the sores to heal faster and prevents the formation of new sores.

2. Famciclovir (Famvir)

Similar to acyclovir, famciclovir is an anti-viral medication that is used to treat the infections caused by certain herpes viruses, most especially herpes zoster. However, for genital herpes outbreak, famciclovir is seen to prevent the onset of future episodes.

3. Valacyclovir (Valtrex)

This drug is very similar with the previous two mentioned anti-viral medications. In addition to what have been mentioned, valacyclovir has also been observed to stop the growth of the virus.

These three pharmaceutical drugs can be all administered as a pill. However, if the symptoms are severe, the doctors usually recommend the intravenous formats of these three medications.

There are times when the patient himself decides to apply some topical meds to relieve the symptoms. It is however being discouraged by many specialist because no benefit or positive effect was observed from the use of topical medications.

There are three treatment interventions for genital herpes. The medications are being given or administered in any of these three phases:

1. Initial treatment

Most patients who consult the help of medical doctors are those whose infections have apparent symptoms. Your doctor will give an antiviral treatment for at least a week in order to relieve the patient of his symptoms. The prescribed medication can also shorten the duration of the symptom outbreak.

If the patient has finished the prescribed medication and still experiencing the same severity of symptoms, the doctor has an option to prescribe the same treatment just with a longer duration.

After the initial treatment, the patient and his doctor might discuss the best antiviral therapy for his condition which could either be suppressive or intermittent treatment.

2. Intermittent treatment

This is a treatment option wherein the doctor will prescribe a set of medications that are designed to control the symptoms upon its first evident signs. The medicines are prescribed to be taken for a set of days in order to control severity of the sores or blisters.

Intermittent medications have also been observed to make the infection to gradually abate.

3. Suppressive treatment

On the other hand, suppressive treatment is designed to those patients who have frequent outbreaks. Doctors advise the patients to take an antiviral drug every day in order to suppress the onset of symptoms. The reduction of outbreak symptoms can be seen at almost 70 to 80%, most especially if you are experiencing 6 to 7 attacks per year.

Doctors have said that there is really no minimum number of onset episodes per year for an individual to avail suppressive medication. The important factor is the onsets are frequent and the attacks are already interfering with the patient's daily life.

Another advantage of suppressive viral medication is the reduction of transferring your infection to your partner. According to a recent study done by valacyclovir, 50% of the people whose partners are infected with HSV didn't contract the disease. Among those who got infected, 75% showed no signs of symptoms.

Safety of Antiviral Medications

As it has been observed, the side effects of the available anti-viral medications are considered to be mild. They all agree that the use of the said drugs is safe even if taken at long term duration. Most of the drugs mentioned have documentations regarding their safety profile and some of them are available in the industry for several years already.

It is advised though that patients under suppressive medication should report to their doctors in order to assess if the treatment is still beneficial or still needed.

Alternative Treatments for Genital Herpes

There are many treatments, both traditional and alternative drugs that have been tested and tried by HSV patients. Among the alternative treatments, there have been winners and there have been losers.

It has been endorsed by numerous patients that the extract of Echinacea plant is instrumental in their ability to fight off the next symptom outbreak. The plant's extract is said to boost the immune system of the patient. Aside from this, it has also been observed to lessen the severity of the symptoms and it can also shorten the duration of the outbreak.

Another alternative medicine that is being used in treating the herpes-related infections is the ointment that contains a substance called propolis. Propolis is a substance that comes from honeybees. Infected people swear that the ointment makes their sores heal faster. This has been tested in a formal study and was indeed confirmed that the ointment with the honeybee-produced substance was effective in healing the sores.

There are some researches that reported the efficacy of an herb named Prunella vulgaris and an edible mushroom called Rozites caperata to be effective in controlling both types of the herpes simplex virus.

New Treatments in the Pipelines

The prevalence of the disease has caused the popularity of herpes simplex virus among drug researchers. As of now, there are numerous new medications already in the pipeline. These medications may either be on their concept or development stage; while some are being tested for side effects, safety and efficacy.

Among these pipeline medications, people are really rooting for a vaccine. However, as of now, results from the tests done were either discouraging or ineffective.

There have also been talks regarding the efficacy of microbicides. Microbicides are chemicals that kill the microbes to prevent infection. This could be used against herpes virus by preventing them from entering the body.

CHAPTER 5 – OUTBREAK PREVENTION AND MANAGEMENT

There are things that you can do in order to prevent the onset of the next symptom outbreak. Several of these things are the following:

a. Friction during sex

There have been some reported cases when it has been observed that the friction during sex is causing irritations to the genital area, thus promoting the onset of sores and blisters.

In such cases, it will be advisable to use a water-based lubricant to help reduce the irritation and to control the friction.

Remember not to use some lubricants other than the water-based types. These lubricants may contain substances like Nonoxynol-9 that is known to irritate the mucous membranes, thus having a good chance to irritate the genital area as well.

Oil based lubricants are also being advised not to be used because such products tend to weaken the elasticity of latex condoms, making them prone to breakage.

b. Colds

Common colds are said to be one of the triggers of the symptom outbreak. However, this may be due to the fact that the immune system of the body is down whenever one has colds.

c. Sunlight

Sunlight exposure are said to be a trigger to HSV1 or cold sores although this has not been taken into formal research or study yet.

d. Hormone changes

Although the mechanism has not been fully known, the hormonal changes that one experiences, like menstrual cycles in females, are said to cause the symptoms to reappear.

e. Surgery and Trauma

When a body experienced a certain injury or trauma, it seems to trigger the nervous system to activate the dormant viruses that live on them. One of the common traumas being experienced by HSV infected patients are surgeries.

f. Weakened immune system

A weakened immune system is the most common trigger of outbreaks. People whose immune systems are compromised by chemotherapy or HIV virus are more likely experience outbreaks than patients without any immunity problems or disorders.

g. Stress

Stress is also one factor seen to cause terrible outbreaks of symptoms.

Stress Management with Genital Herpes

Stress is one of factors that trigger the onset of HSV symptoms. This is why it is crucial to avoid it as much as possible. What you can do is to find ways to manage your stress.

The following items are guidelines that can help you in stress management:

1. Sleep with enough hours

Sleep is the body's reboot and it can do wonders to our body and health. Enough hours of sleep can give you more acuity to handle your problems well without producing any stress-related complications.

2. Balanced diet

You have to watch out some foods that trigger stress. Some of these are coffee and alcohol. Pile some fruits and vegetables in order to refresh your body and internal systems.

3. Exercise

It has been said before and has been proven many times over to relieve stress. Do a physical activity that you honestly enjoy. This way, it would not feel like you are obliged to do the physical exercise.

4. Socialize

Be with people whose company you enjoy and

surround yourself with friends. Episodes of laughter can very well prevent you from ever thinking the matter that makes you stressed and tensed in the first place.

5. Relax

Breathe and make yourself feel rested even only for a while. A rest can do you good if you are constantly slaving yourself to work.

CHAPTER 6 – COPING WITH GENITAL HERPES DIAGNOSIS

Hearing the words of your doctor confirming that you are indeed infected with HSV2 is not very easy to take. A virus with no cure is not really the kind of gift you wanted to get from your partner.

However, the reality will really have to be accepted and it is advised that you learn how to live with it because the virus will of course stay with you for the rest of your years.

First, what you need to do is to accept it. You can only do something about it if you are convinced that you really have it. Bear in mind that it is not the end of the world. There are still effective things that you can do in order to suppress the outbreaks and the painful and sometimes embarrassing symptoms.

Second, you will have to tell yourself that you cannot be condemned just because of such illness. There are ways in which you cannot infect your partner. You just have to make sure that you would not engage with sex if you have symptoms.

You also have to learn to live with pills. There are also some diseases and conditions that require maintenance pills and herpes simplex viral infection are not an exemption.

A FINAL WORD

I want to take this time out to thank you for purchasing this book! The next step is to take action on the advice you've just read about.

Please Leave a Review

Finally, if you enjoyed this book, please take the time to share your thoughts and post a review on Amazon. It'd be greatly appreciated!

That review and feedback will help me improve the content in my books – and make each and every one more relevant and helpful to you.

Thank you again and good luck!

Angie S

www.ingramcontent.com/pod-product-compliance
Lightning Source LLC
Chambersburg PA
CBHW070240290526
45789CB00004B/1700
* 9 7 8 1 4 9 9 5 3 9 5 9 2 *